Allopathy and Homoeopathy

Before the Judgment of Common Sense

Published by Thirty-Three & 1/3⅓ Publishing, LLC

ISBN-13: 978-1974675746

ISBN-10: 1974675742

First published San Francisco: Bruce's Job Printing House, 535 Sacramento Street, 1872), Author Frederick Hiller, M.D

Copyright © Published by

Thirty-Three & 1/3⅓ Publishing, LLC., 2017

All Rights Reserved.

Printed and bound in the United States of America

Transcriber's note: Hyphenation and spelling have been retained as in the original. Both "household" and "house-hold" were used in the original; unusually spelled words include: practitoners, peurile, unwaranted, brigther and recieved.

The oe-ligature is represented by the letters oe enclosed in brackets ([oe]).

ALLOPATHY AND HOMOEOPATHY

Before the Judgment of Common Sense!

by

F. HILLER, M.D.

It is difficult to carry the Torch-Light of Truth through the masses, without stepping occasionally upon a toe or burning a wig or a head-dress.

To WILLIAM SHARON, Esq., ISAAC L. REQUA, Esq., A. K. P. HARMON, Esq., SAMUEL G. THELLER, Esq. GENTLEMEN: I have taken the liberty to dedicate this offering to you, as a token of respect and esteem. This, together with a grateful remembrance of the courtesies extended to me, and the support which I have derived from your friendship, will be, I hope, a sufficient excuse for the liberty I have taken. Very truly, yours, etc.

Allopathy and Homoeopathy Before the by Frederick Hiller

F. HILLER, M.D. San Francisco, 1872.

TO THE MEMORY OF

SAMUEL HAHNEMANN

THE DISCOVERER OF

THE TRUE LAW OF CURE

Born April 10th, 1775

Died June 4th, 1843.

LADIES AND GENTLEMEN:

It is a remarkable and at the same time a terrible and most lamentable fact, that the practice of medicine--an art of daily necessity and application, most nearly affecting the dearest interests and well being of mankind, and to the improvement of which we are encouraged and impelled by the strongest motives of interest and humanity, of love for our neighbor and emulous zeal for professional skill and superiority therein--should, after a probation of so long a period, and recorded experience of at least two thousand years, still remain, as it confessedly does in most respects, so little understood and generally of such doubtful and uncertain application.

The present age, unlike any that has preceded it, is peculiarly one of rigid, radical and fundamental examination. Everything in the Heavens above, or in the Earth beneath, is tested and retested; analyzed, synthetized and submitted to the crucible of stern reason, and the logical conclusion of experience; even to the extreme of possibility. This is true not only of the material universe, but of all mental and moral conditions, of social, political and even religious institutions. Nothing, in this day, and especially in this country of free thought and liberty of speech, is taken for granted merely because it can lay claim to the honors of a great antiquity, or can number thousands or millions of adherents. Vast differences are to be observed in governments, churches, creeds and social practices; and all, however opposite and apparently antagonistic, are working out a solution to the problem--

"WHAT IS TRUTH?"

Conservatism is fast dying out, hidden and smothered by the ever-flowing tidal-waves of progression. Radicalism ceases to become radical, by the daily and hourly recurrence of startling discoveries, and new, unheard-of, and unexpected adaptations of old laws. The mistakes of to-day will be found to be mistakes, and will be rectified. Whenever and wherever freedom holds her sway, evil must work out its own destruction, and good enthrone itself in the hearts of those benefitted by its benign influence. In this spirit, and with such views, let us look at the progress of Medical Science that we may learn from the experience of the past to correctly estimate the developments of the present and aid wisely in the working for a more glorious future.

Medicine has been--not inaptly styled--"The daughter of dreams." From the time of Hippocrates until now, the great body of the profession has been swayed by conflicting theories, founded upon either the wholly unsupported fancies and conjectures of their authors, or unwarrantably built upon isolated facts, often accidental in their occurence, partial in their observation, and improperly understood in their inherent nature and theoretical significance, pointing to a law of action widely different from the one in support of which they had been adduced. All branches of medicine have been involved in these crude absurdities; nor has the nomenclature of any department of science, even in our day, been entirely purged from the errors and misleadings with which the past so fruitfully abounds.

To mark the improvement and advancement in the various branches of medical science; to compare the present with the past; to observe the unfolding growth, maturity, and decay of medical creeds; to discern the power of those master-minds, that, far beyond the ages in which they lived foreshadowed the forth-coming discoveries that were to make other men immortal; to sigh over the incredulity of whole races, whose blind and dogmatical adherence to the theories of some prominent physiologist or anatomist--was at once silenced by the light of a new truth, suddenly and clearly promulgated by a single mind. To do all these things, was the labor of a whole life; volumes could be written in such investigation, and still thousands of facts be left untouched and forgotten, forever buried in the chaos of medical creeds, medical truths and medical fictions.

Old Physic has for several centuries past drifted in the wrong direction, striking occasionally upon a rock, but finds itself to day further off from shore than ever before.

Medicine, the oldest and most important of all branches of science, has not kept up with developments in other departments, but the rays of light have already deeply penetrated into the darkness of the past, fast undermining the building of the so-called "Rational Medicine" with all its hypothesis and traditions.

* * * * *

It was near the end of the last century, that the idea occurred to a single man, that the reason he had failed in practice must be that the medical profession was entirely on the wrong path. He made the effort to cure diseases on the principle directly opposite to those on which he had been educated to act, and he was successful. He thought a reformation of medicine needful and desirable, and proper to be attempted. He set about it, hoping, if he should succeed in pointing out a more safe, certain and pleasant road to the life-giving and life-renewing fountain of health, that it would be a blessing to suffering humanity. That man was SAMUEL HAHNEMANN.

Had the reform inaugurated by him been of an insignificant character, it might have been accepted by the medical world without controversy. Had the new path into which he invited the profession been only a little smoother than the old one and lying right alongside of it, like that which led the pilgrims from the main high-way into the domains of the giant, physicians might have been easily lured into it. But the revolution was a radical one. It contemplated a countermarch such as the teachers and practitoners of the healing art had never been called upon to make. It called upon the chiefs of the profession to reverse the wheels of the ponderous engine, and seek for the long-sought shore in the opposite direction.

The new doctrine came forth embodied in only three simple words: "Similia Similibus Curantur."

Thus the year 1790 gave birth to the

celebrated system of Hahnemann, which has received from him a Greek title, expressive of its peculiarities--Hom[oe]opathy, and in opposition to "Contraria Contraries Curantur."--Allopathy.

It is not my purpose to entertain you with a detailed history of medicine, nor even to notice the successive and conflicting theories that have arisen from time to time; but simply to show that the old, or Allopathic system of medicine as practiced till this day is unworthy of our confidence; that its theory of therapeutics is irrational and worthless; that there is an absence of any reliable principle to guide the physicians in the treatment of diseases; and that the sick are far better off when left to nature, than when subject to the pernicious system of dosing, while a growing want of confidence in this system, both in the public mind and the medical profession, loudly calls for something more rational in its theory and more successful in its practice.

I shall not ask you to accept my individual opinions in support of these views, but shall place upon the witness-stand, and give you the declarations of men who have spent their lives in the practice of this system-- most of them authors and teachers, men living in different countries, and from the highest ranks of the profession, and who, if any, should be able to pronounce a eulogy upon this system of practice.

I introduce to you first BOERHAVE, a man justly illustrious in the history of medicine, he lived a century before HAHNEMANN, and was for over forty years Professor at the University at Leiden.

Hear him! He says:

"If we compare the good which a half dozen true disciples of Æsculapius have done since their art began, with the evil which the immense number of doctors have inflicted upon mankind, we must be satisfied that it would have been infinitely better for mankind if medical men had never existed."

The celebrated BICHAT of Paris, thus speaks of the therapeutic system of his day:

"It is an incoherent assemblage of incoherent opinions; it is perhaps, of all the physiological sciences that which best shows the caprice of the human mind. What do I say?--It is not a science for a methodical mind; it is a shapeless assemblage of inexact ideas, of observations often peurile, of deceptive remedies and of formula as fastidiously and fantastically conceived, as they are tediously arranged."

Then we find the equally celebrated French physician, MAJENDIE, saying:

"I hesitate not to declare, no matter how sorely I shall wound our vanity, that so gross is our ignorance of the physiological disorders called diseases, that it would perhaps be better to do nothing, and resign the complaint we are called upon to treat to the resources of Nature, than to act as we frequently do, without knowing the why and the wherefore of our conduct, and at the obvious risk of hastening the end of our patient."

DR. GOOD, the great nosologist, asserts that

"The science of medicine is a barbarous jargon, and the effects of our medicines on the human system are in the highest degree uncertain; except, indeed, that they have already destroyed more lives than war, pestilence and famine combined."

SIR ASTLEY COOPER, England's greatest surgeon says:

"The science of medicine is founded on conjecture and improved by murder."

But, it may be said, these men lived in the past, and since their time the science of medicine has improved and its practice has become more rational and safe.

* * * * *

Let us then come down to a later period, and listen to DR. CHRISTISON, the present eminent Professor of Materia Medica at the University of Edinburgh. He says:

"Of all medical sciences, therapeutics is the most unsatisfactory in its present state, and the least advanced in progress, and surrounded by the most deceitful sources of fallacy."

SIR JOHN FORBES, Fellow of the Royal College of Physicians: Physician to the Queen's Household, late

editor of the "British and Foreign Medical Review," after a frank admission of the imperfections of Allopathic medicine, says:

"FIRST. That in a large proportion of the cases treated by Allopathic physicians, the disease is cured by Nature and not by them."

"SECOND. That in a lesser, but still not a small proportion, the disease is cured in spite of them; in other words, their interference opposing instead of assisting the cure."

"THIRD. That, consequently in a considerable proportion of diseases, it would be as well, or better with patients, in the actual condition of the medical art, as more generally practiced, if all remedies, at least active remedies especially drugs were abandoned." And finally adds, "Things have arrived at such a pitch that they cannot be worse. They must mend or end."

But, I may be asked, what are the views of the Professors and writers in our own country. Have they no more confidence in the healing art than their brethren in the old world? Let us see:

DR. RUSH, one of the lights of the profession in his day, remarks:

"The healing art is an unroofed temple,

uncovered at the top and cracked at the foundation."

And again:

"Our want of success results from the following causes: FIRST.--Ignorance of the law governing disease. SECOND.--Our ignorance of a suitable remedy THIRD.--Want of efficacy in the remedy; and finally we have assisted in multiplying disease; nay, we have done more: we have increased their mortality."

Professor CHAPMAN, who stood at the head of the profession in Philadelphia, in an address to the medical society, after speaking of the pernicious effects of calomel, adds:

"Gentlemen, it is a disgraceful reproach to the profession of medicine; it is quackery, horrid unwaranted murderous quackery.... But I will ask another question, who is it that can stop the career of mercury at will, after it has taken the reins into its own destructive and ungovernable hands? He, who for an ordinary cause resigns the fate of his patient to mercury is a vile enemy to the sick; and if he is tolerably popular, will, in one successful season, have paved the way for the business of life, for he has enough to do ever afterwards to stop the mercurial breach of the constitutions of his dilapidated patients."

And yet, this article of the Materia Medica in some of its various forms, is still more frequently prescribed than any other by the allopathic physicians. A writer in the June number, 1868, of the "London Chemist," having submitted to a careful examination one thousand prescriptions, taken seriatim from the files of a druggist, states, among other curious facts, that mercury takes the lead, and stands prominently at the head of the list. Mercury, the very name of which strikes terror into the minds of nervous and timid patients, is still the foremost remedial agent employed by the medical profession.

Professor DRAPER, in one of his introductory lectures, before the University College of New York, makes the following statement:

"Even those of us who have most carefully upheld our old professional theories, and have tried to keep in reverence the old opinions, and the old times, find that under the advance of the exact sciences our position is becoming untenable. The ground is slipping away from beneath our feet. We are on the brink of a great revolution. Go where you will, among intelligent physicians you will find a deep, though it may be an indistinct perception, that a great change is imminent."

The late Professor MUTTER of Philadelphia, in an introductory lecture a few years ago, says:

"We have in truth, rested contented in ideal knowledge. We have received as perfect, theories as idle as day dreams. We have blindly accepted the follies of the past; and the foundation of our art must crumble to the earth unless we learn more discretion and better judgment in the selection of the material of which they are to be constructed."

I might continue these quotations indefinitely; but I will not weary you by citing more, and surely, sufficient evidence has already been produced to sustain the allegation that the old system of medicine is unworthy of our confidence; that, with no law upon which to base its principles of treatment, its practice rests upon a chaotic mass of empirical experiences, groundless theories, and ever-changing fancies; that those best acquainted with its principles, and the results of its practice, have the least faith in its usefulness; and that the interests of the suffering, imperiously demand a revolution in the method of treating disease, and call for a system more in harmony with Nature, more reliable in its application, and more successful in its results.

This degraded state of the medical practice was deeply felt by HAHNEMANN, and in 1778 he retired from the practice of medicine in disgust at its uncertainties, after having acquired fame as a scientific scholar and high standing in his profession, breaking away from the past and opening a new field of glory to his activities, as well as a new era of progress in the medical art.

SAMUEL HAHNEMANN was a great man; the discoverer of the true law of cure, in accordance with the principles and laws of Nature.

I need not tell you, that we maintain that this much-desired and long-looked-for law of cure, which is to be a lamp to the feet of the physician, making plain his path, and giving him an unfailing guide in the application of remedies to the removal of disease, not only exists, but has been proclaimed to the world by the immortal Hahnemann in his well-known formula: Similia Similibus Curantur!

But who was Samuel Hahnemann? When I say that this great Reformer of Medicine was a regularly educated physician of great learning and unusual general culture and literary attainments, I speak but feeble praise compared with the language of Sir John Forbes, Hahnemann's most learned critic, where he says:

"No candid reader of his writings can hesitate for a moment to admit that he was a very extraordinary man; one, whose name will descend to posterity as the exclusive excogitator and founder of an original system of medicine, as ingenious as many that preceded it, and destined to be the remote, if not the immediate cause of more fundamental changes in the practice of the healing art, than have resulted from any promulgated since the days of GALEN himself."

And he adds:

"He was undoubtedly a man of genius and a scholar, a man of indefatigable industry and of dauntless energy."

The great HALLER, says of him:

"He is a doublehead of philosophy and wisdom."

And HUFELAND, the father of orthodox medicine, speaks of him as one of the most distinguished physicians in Germany, while the late DR. MOTT of New York, after having visited HAHNEMANN in Paris, speaks in the highest terms of his candor, learning and genius.

It has often been stated by close observers of the working of Divine Providence, that

"The darkest hour is just before day," and also, that "The Creator ever wisely and well provides agents perfectly adapted to carry out His beneficent designs in the crisis of human affairs." History, both sacred and profane, gives unwavering and very numerous evidences of the justice and verity of these propositions. In matters theological as well as political this is equally the case. When there could scarcely be greater gloom or greater danger, the wise Arbiter of human destinies has educated, nerved, inspired and protected some master-spirit, who has caused light to shine out of darkness, and peace and order to take the place of chaos and destruction. Never were these propositions more fully illustrated than in medical matters towards the close of the past century. All the arts and sciences had received the impetus of new discoveries.

The inductive method of investigation had brought out clearly to view first principles, on which it was easy for succeeding generations to build solid, stable and beautiful temples of truth.

Astronomy, chemistry, botany and every branch in Natural Philosophy, instead of continuing mere matters of speculative theory, as they were before, became sciences. The sons of Æsculapius alone were enshrouded in an Egyptian darkness, wandering about without guide and compass, rushing wildly to and fro with instruments of deadly power in their hands; whom they wished to heal, they slew; and tortured those whom they fondly hoped might find timely relief from sufferings and woes through their ministrations.

The hearts of the benevolent were deeply

pained, and the conscientious wavered in their work when they gathered statistics of the results of their labor. A cry ascended heaven-wards from the practitioners of medicine, the longing for better days, seemed seconded by a phalanx of ghostly beings, who had untimely passed away by means of fearful treatment, and by the living miseries of multitudes of shapeless deformed ones, who ever stood unpleasant and incontrovertible witnesses of the cruelties and barbarities of the healing art.

With increasing civilization, new and fatal epidemics appeared, reaping a rich harvest for the grim monster--Death--and adding yearly to the per-centage of the ever-increasing bills of mortality. Many an honest practitioner threw away lancet and saddle-bags in despair, while quacks and medical charlatans, profiting by the wranglings of the regulars, and the weariness of the people, drove a reckless but well-paying trade, with nostrums of every character, from the deadliest poison to the simplest house-hold herb.

BUT A BRIGTHER DAY WAS ABOUT TO DAWN.

In the picturesque town of Meissen, in the district of Cur Saxony, lived an honest and worthy man, Christian Gottfried Hahnemann, an intelligent, patriotic and highly esteemed, though unassuming and unambitious member of that community, by trade a painter upon porcelain, known under the name of Dresden-China.

On the 10th day of April, 1755, he was made happy by the birth of a son, whom he named

Samuel Christian Frederick. Amidst all the fond hopes the parents cherished for their new-born babe, little did they imagine to what a destiny the great Creator had appointed him. Of the mother of this child not very much is known, save that she was modest, industrious, intensely attached to her family, full of sympathy with her children's aspirations, and ever-ready to aid them in their schemes of pleasure or advancement. The infantile years of little Hahnemann were spent amidst scenery so strikingly beautiful, as to impress his young buoyant heart, even in those tender years, with an admiration of Nature's handiwork, and so instill into him a love of the works of God, which ever increased as he grew older. He was not sent to school very young, not until he was eight years old; this will perhaps partly account for the fact that when he did go, he manifested an ardent thirst for knowledge, which was never slacked during his long life-time. But he did not spend his first eight years of life entirely in play. Those health-securing, physical-exhilarating and developing exercises were occasionally relieved by lessons from his father, and sometimes from his mother, in reading and writing, and by frequent conversations of a religious and moral character.

These conversations laid deep the foundation of that undeviating integrity, fixedness of purpose, unwavering conscientiousness and unaffected reverence for the Divine Being, which ever characterized this Medical Reformer in after life. The influence of this paternal conversational instruction and moral training made him what he was, as a school-boy, as a college-student, as an author, a chemist and a physician. Untiring industry, conscientiousness, and a reliance upon Divine blessing, will in any sphere in life secure success, and Samuel Hahnemann was no exception to the general rule. In writing on this subject, he says: "My father had the soundest ideas on what was to be considered good and worthy in man, and had arrived at them by his own independent thought. He sought to plant them in me, and impressed on me more by actions than by words, the great lesson of life, to act and to be, not merely to seem! When a good work was going forward, there, often unobserved, he was sure to be helping, hand to heart; shall I not do likewise? In the finest distinctions between the noble and the base, he decided by his actions with a justness that did honor to the nicety of his sense of right and wrong. In this, too, he was my monitor."

Such sterling qualities, rooted in the boy's heart, and early budding out in his life, made him beloved by all who came in contact with him. Play-mates, school-fellows and instructors not only treated him with kindness, but with ardent affection.

This school-boy life did not pass, however, without trials, the greatest of which was the disinclination of his father for him to continue his studies. It is a little strange that the good man, who himself possessed a keen power of observation, did not once suspect the future greatness of his child: but he was very poor, had several other children to support, and doubtless feared that a thorough classical and scientific education would give to his son aspirations that would be doomed to bitter disappointment. His teacher, however, pleaded on his behalf, offering to remit the usual school-fees, and he was permitted to continue his studies until he was twenty years of age. A proof of the poverty of his parents at this time, is illustrated by the circumstance, that his father complained of the great consumption of oil during young Hahnemann's preparation of his lessons, and would not permit him to use the family lamp after the other members of the household had retired: but Samuel, who was never daunted by difficulties, or frustrated in a purpose, when he had concluded that it was legitimate, manufactured a lamp out of a lump of clay, and successfully coaxed his mother to supply him with oil.

At the close of his high school term, young Hahnemann wrote, as was usual with those just finishing their course, a treatise. He had for some time manifested a deep interest in natural science, and particularly in the branches of chemistry and physiology. He wrote his thesis in Latin, choosing as his subject, "The wisdom of God in forming the Human Hand." This was for his age, a work of great merit, and even his father seemed to have become proud of his abilities, and gave his free consent for the studious boy to go to Leipzig that he might attend the lectures at the University, and presented him with all the money he possibly could spare, amounting to nearly fifteen dollars in our currency. "This," says Hahnemann, "was the last money I received from my father." He left his home for Leipzig on Easter, 1775.

He was at first somewhat puzzled by that troublesome subject, "the ways and means," but fortunately becoming acquainted with two rich Princes of Greece, who were anxious to be instructed in the English and French languages. Hahnemann entered into a lucrative engagement with them as instructor, and also obtained employment as a translator of medical and philosophical works. The remuneration he received for private teaching and translating, not only enabled him to supply all his moderate wants and purchase of books, but he saved a considerable amount besides. In order to save so much, and at the same time attend faithfully upon all his classes, he denied himself sleep every other night. In 1777, we find him attending the hospitals of Vienna where his excellence of character, and extent of medical information, completely won him the friendship and confidence of the celebrated Doctor von Quarin, who perceiving the noble qualities and promising abilities of the young man, adopted him as a special protégé. Hahnemann says of him, "To him I owe my claims to be reckoned as a physician. I had his love and friendship." After this, he visited the University of Erlangen, where he graduated, receiving the degree of Doctor of Medicine on the 10th of August, 1779. At this time, an earnest longing for the air of Saxony and the scenery of his native district seems to have taken possession of him. After having occupied several prominent positions, the government offered him the office of District Physician in Gommern, which he accepted in 1782.

After three years residence in Gommern, during which time he had married, he became tired of professional

idleness--as he expresses himself--and we

find him removing to Dresden. For about a year he occupied the position as superintendent of the public hospitals of that city. His conscience however, began to be much troubled by the conviction that medicine as then practiced proved worse than useless to the majority of patients. He retired from the practice of medicine in disgust at its uncertainties, occupying himself solely with chemistry and literary labor.

* * * * *

The humanity and integrity of Hahnemann is plainly portrayed in a letter to the venerable Hufeland, where he gives his own account of the reasons which induced him at this time to retire from practice. He writes:

"It was painful for me to grope in the dark,

guided only by our books in the treatment of the sick--to prescribe according to this or that fanciful view of the nature of diseases, substances that only owed to mere opinion their place in the Materia Medica. I had conscientious scruples about treating unknown morbid states in my suffering fellow-creatures with these unknown medicines; which, being powerful substances, might, if they were not exactly suitable, (and how could the physician know whether they were suitable or not, seeing that their peculiar special actions were not yet elucidated?), easily change life into death, or produce new affections or chronic ailments, which are often much more difficult to remove than the original disease. To become in this way a murderer, or an aggravator of the sufferings of mankind, was to me a fearful thought. So fearful and distressing was it, that shortly after my marriage I abandoned the practice, and scarcely treated any one for fear of doing him harm."

In 1789, he settled in Leipzig, and numerous writings and translations, which have been often quoted by the best writers ever since, came from his pen during that period. We come now to the year 1790, in which the first thought of Hom[oe]opathy issued from the brain of the great father and founder of the new school of medicine. It has already been hinted that Hahnemann had felt an intense desire to obtain some clear, safe and philosophical guide to the therapeutic action of drugs.

He was called upon to translate "Cullen's Materia Medica," and as he progressed in the description of one medical substance after another, he could not but feel a renewal of the earnest longing he had so often cherished, to clear medical science from the clouds of mist and uncertainty in which it had continued from the time of Hippocrates.

✷ ✷ ✷ ✷ ✷

The workings of his mind, and the character of the man, at this time will be best understood by a quotation from the letter he wrote to Hufeland, where he says:

"Having briefly reviewed, the sad experience of the systems of Sydenham and Hoffmann, of Boerhave and Glaubius, of Stahl, Cullen and de Hean," he continues,

"But it is, perhaps, the very nature of this art, as great men have asserted that it is incapable of attaining any greater certainty. Shameful, blasphemous thought! What! shall it be said that the infinite wisdom of the Eternal Spirit, that animates the universe, could not produce remedies to allay the sufferings of the diseases He allows to arise? The all-loving paternal goodness of Him, whom no name worthily designates, who richly supplies all wants, even the scarcely conceivable wants of the insect in the dust, imperceptible by reason of its minuteness to the keenest human eye, and who despenses throughout creation, life and happiness in rich abundance, shall it be said that He is capable of the tyranny of not permitting that man, made in his image, should by the efforts of his penetrating mind, that has been breathed into him from above, find out the way to discover remedies in the stupendous kingdom of creation, which should be able to deliver mankind from their sufferings, worse than death itself? Shall He, the Father of all, behold with indifference the martyrdom of his best-beloved creatures by disease, and yet render it impossible to the genius of man, to whom all else is possible, to find any method, any easy, sure, trust-worthy method, whereby they may see diseases from their proper point of view, and whereby they may interrogate medicines as to their special uses, as to what they are really, surely and positively serviceable for? Well, thought I, as there must be a sure and trust-worthy method of treatment, as certainly as God is the wisest and most beneficient of Beings, I shall seek it no longer in the thorny thicket of ontological explanations,... nor in the authoritative declarations of celebrated men. No; let me seek it where it lies nearest at hand, and where it has hitherto been passed over by all, because it did not seem sufficiently recondite, nor sufficiently learned, and was not hung with laurels for those who displayed most talent for constructing systems, for scholastic speculation, and transcendental abstractions."

With these high and noble feelings, his mind was fully awake to any suggestion that might be derived from the material before him.

For forty years he carried on a series of well-planned and well-calculated experiments to ascertain the disease-producing power of drugs, when administered to persons in health. Friends, medical and lay, were brought into requisition, and all possible means taken to secure the greatest accuracy; for Hahnemann already began to feel that he was God's agent of mercy, through whose happy discovery and labors future generations would be greatly blessed.

He found but little opportunity to test his newly-discovered law of cure while he remained in Leipzig, and poverty compelled him to labor with his pen most indefatigably, as was evidenced by the large number of essays and translations published at that time.

Providence, however, interfered in his behalf; the reigning Duke of Saxe Gotha offered him the position of Physician to the Asylum for the Insane in Georgenthal, in the Thuringen Forest. He entered upon his duties in 1792. While at the head of this establishment, he succeeded in affecting a cure which created some sensation, because the party concerned was the Hanoverian Minister, Klockenbring, who was rendered insane by a lampoon written by Kotzebue. He also introduced a mild and humane treatment for the insane, removing the chains and tight-jacket, heretofore in use.

In 1810, he published his greatest work, "The Organon," which ran through five editions, and was translated into most all the living languages. From 1810 to 1821, we find him again in Leipzig, publishing his Materia Medica, and lecturing twice a week in the University, at the same time attending to a multitude of patients.

In 1821, Hahnemann was induced by the reigning Duke of Anhalt-Coethen, who was his warm friend and admirer, to change his place of residence, and appointed him his Physician. He accepted the position. He soon began to work as earnestly as before in proving medicines and prescribing for his patients, who came from all parts of Europe.

On one occasion, during his residence in Coethen, he recieved a visitor who had heard a great deal of Hahnemann and his garden, and who had imagined the garden to be as large as its owner was great. When he was ushered into the presence of the Prophet of Medicine and found him seated at a table in a summer-house, only a few yards from the dwelling, he exclaimed: "But where is the garden?" To which Hahnemann replied, "This is the garden." "Surely," rejoined the visitor, "Not this narrow patch of ground?" "True, it is very narrow and very short, but observe its infinite height," said the Sage, pointing upwards to the blue sky overhead.

The tenth of August, 1829, was a joyful day for the venerable old man, being the fifteenth anniversary of his obtaining the degree of M. D. Gratifying and memorable in more than one respect was this day for him.

I refrain from giving you a full description of this impressive celebration, lest I should be considered tedious, yet I cannot thus pass over historical facts, without dwelling upon a few of the principal features of this gratifying and memorable festivity.

The early morning found assembled a large number of the friends of Hahnemann, his disciples; deputations from various cities; also deputations from the Universities of Leipzig, Vienna and Erlangen, which presented him with the Diploma of Honor. The King of Saxony, the Duke of Saxe Gotha and many others had sent costly presents from far and near. His dwelling having been appropriately prepared for the celebration, and on a table, resembling an altar, adorned with flowers and entwined with oak leaves, was placed a well executed bust of

Hahnemann.

After Hahnemann was introduced, his bust was crowned with laurels, amid appropriate addresses and congratulations. With deep emotion, the venerable old man in heartfelt and affecting words, gave thanks to the Supreme Being that he had been permitted to make so great a discovery, and was so favored with a long life, full of bodily and mental vigor.

A year after this important occurrence, the Asiatic Cholera came marching from the East, for the first time. This aroused the medical profession in general. Physicians were helpless, and none of them had ever seen a case of this fearful disease. But Hahnemann, after learning the symptoms of the disease, advised the mode of treatment by which the mortality of that terrible scourge was threefold reduced, and numerous testimonials were published, showing the immense success of his mode of treatment. In 1831, he lost his partner in life, having been married forty-nine years and a few months.

About four years after the death of his wife, a most interesting, intelligent and estimable lady, applied to Hahnemann for advice for lung and heart disease. It has been humorously stated that though the lung disease was effectually cured, the trouble of the heart must have assumed a chronic form, for the fascinating Parisienne seemed deeply enamored with the great doctor. She was 35 years of age, the daughter of Louis Jerome Cohier, formerly Minister of Justice and President and Director of the French Republic, her name was Marie Melanie d'Herville Cohier. This lady of position and wealth offered her hand to the octogenarian, which he accepted, and after having divided his considerable fortune among his children, upon which his young wife insisted, he was induced by her to pass the rest of his life in Paris, where he enjoyed a great reputation till his death, which took place July 2nd, 1843. On the centenary of his birthday in 1855, a statute was erected to his memory at Leipzig.

* * * * *

To complete the picture of this great man, I have to cite from a letter written by Dr. Jahr in Paris on the fourth of July 1843, where he says:

"Hahnemann is dead! In fact, dear friends, our venerable father had finished his career. A pulmonary paralysis had set him free, after an illness of six weeks, finally liberating the great soul from its earthly tenement. To the last moment, he was in the possession of his mental faculties.... In the commencement of that illness he announced that it would be his last, as his body was worn out. At first he prescribed for himself, and nearly to the period of his death delivered his opinion of the remedies offered him by his wife and Dr. Chartran.... When his wife, on account of a fit of suffocation, said to him, 'Providence ought to exempt you from these sufferings, as you have relieved so many, and endured such numerous persecutions,' he replied, 'Me: why me? Every one works according to the abilities and powers which Providence has bestowed upon him. Superiority or inferiority exists only before the tribunal of men, not before that of Providence. Providence owes nothing to me, but I am indebted to Providence for all.'"

I leave these memorable words, for every one to deduce from them the natural conclusion, and especially as truly illustrative of the character of Hahnemann. The grand old man, at 80 years of age, launched himself upon a new career in the capital of

France. In three years we find him making an income of 200,000 francs a year from his professional exertions, and giving gratuitous advice to crowds of the poor.

Year after year his wonderful successes brought him a rapid increase to even this large income. In his 89th year he died and left a fortune of 4,000,000 francs, nearly a million of dollars.

Seldom has a man ended his days in so glorious a sunset, or in a surer hope for the future.

The merit of Hahnemann, and that for which we ought to bless his name and cherish his memory, is his rejection of theory and the establishment of the curative art upon the solid foundation of science. All that was merely speculative he rejected as unsafe, and sought by pure experiment and objective observation, to find out Nature's law of cure. Taking nothing for truth that could not be proved by experiment, he, by careful and untiring observation, obtained from Nature the answer that Similia Similibus Curantur was the law of cure, the only scientific law to heal disease.

This science is not wafted to and fro by the winds of opinion and supposition. It is through its organic unity, as firm and unchanging as Nature itself. In it all medical men must agree, because the reign of supposition has been replaced by that of facts, and all animated by the spirit of progress will work actively and earnestly in promoting science and the art of healing for their own benefit, and that of suffering humanity in general. To get such a science recognized and spread over the world, is undoubtedly a noble problem of the age. Hahnemann also discovered by experiment and pure objective observation, that disease renders the organization wonderfully sensitive to their specific remedies, so that the mere smell of the specific drug can, in many cases effect a cure; and that in all cases, a very small dose of the true remedy is all that is required; so small as to have no effect whatever on the organism in a state of health; and further, that large doses, even of the proper remedy, are not only useless, but hurtful, being calculated to aggravate the disease and endanger vitality.

Time will not permit me to attempt here an elucidation of the principles and doctrines promulgated by Hahnemann; yet I wish to notice briefly some of the results following the introduction of Hom[oe]opathy into the medical world. It is now about seventy-five years since Hahnemann made public, and taught this new system of medicine. The bold reformer and his disciples were persecuted, ridiculed and scorned in every manner by the so-called orthodox doctors, who declared their principles so ridiculous and nonsensical, that it would be below the dignity of a scientific man to make himself acquainted with the laws and practice of Hom[oe]opathy. But Hom[oe]opathy in the theoretical and practical proofs of its universal importance, deserves to be ranked among the most important discoveries of the age, and as one of the most beneficial discoveries that humanity has ever been blessed with.

Men of the highest standing in the

profession have given their unqualified indorsement of its foundation as an indisputable law of Nature, and of its right to be considered high in the order of science.

The truth of its principles has been practically proven by its success, not only in isolated cases, but in great epidemics, as those of dysentery, cholera, yellow fever, typhus, smallpox, scarlet fever, measles, diptheria, etc.; and this, too, in so conspicuous a manner, that year after year, it has forced its way into larger and higher circles, and is now practiced in all countries by a large number of scientific and intelligent physicians, who, after having studied and practiced for a longer or shorter length of time the murderous system of Allopathy, are acquainted with both, and have given the preference to

Hom[oe]opathy, only after mature reflection, investigation and numerous comparisons of the result of both systems in their practice.

The great majority of Old-School physicians, only know Hom[oe]opathy by hearsay, and look upon it through the dim glasses of the prejudices of the past. None of those who have abused Hom[oe]opathy have previously examined and studied the matter thoroughly, because all those who have conscientiously done this, have soon been converted to the truth of the system and have adopted its practice.

In the ranks of the practitioners and believers in Hom[oe]opathy, we see physicians whose writings prove, and to whom nobody can deny an extended and profound medical knowledge, as well as judgment. Hom[oe]opathy can boast of a rich and scientific literature, and a great number of profound writings in all the languages of the civilized world.

Hom[oe]opathy is a vast and steadily growing power in the medical and scientific world, demanding earnestly the attention of every intelligent man. Its real merit may be partially measured by the strength of obstacles it has had to overcome.

Hom[oe]opathy is a reform in the central and main field of medical practice, a reform effected by the discovery of a great and true therapeutic law, and by the construction of a new Materia Medica, which reveals to us the disease-producing properties of drugs. It has rendered pathology the highest service by making that great branch of medical science truly practical; for, an exact parallel functional and organic law between the phenomena of diseases and drugs is necessary to the scientific selection of hom[oe]opathic medicines. By its great therapeutic law, it has introduced new light, order, beauty and efficiency into the theory and practice of medicine. It has cured thousands of cases of chronic disease, beyond the reach of allopathic art, and has treated all acute diseases with admirable ease and success. In great epidemics, it proved always superior to the old system. I was converted by experiencing the wonderful effects of hom[oe]opathic medicine on myself, but particularly by witnessing the triumphs of Hom[oe]opathy in the treatment of the Asiatic cholera, in the terrible epidemic of 1849-'50 and '51.

Allopathic mortality was 56 per c.

Hom[oe]opathic mortality was 12 per c.

In yellow fever, its success was equally surprising. Drs. Davis and Holcombe treated over a thousand cases at Natchez in 1853 and '55, with a mortality of 7 per cent. Allopathy lost two-thirds of its patients. On account of this great victory, they were elected physicians and surgeons of the Mississippi State Hospital, which was till then under allopathic government. The reports from that Institution are triumphs to Hom[oe]opathy up to the present day, and confirmatory of the superiority of this system of medical treatment.

Hom[oe]opathy has saved thousands of cases from surgical operations, and has introduced safety into the lying-in-room of woman. It has been a blessing to children, and to mothers incalculably beneficial. It has been found equally useful in the diseases of animals, and many veterinary institutions have been established for its practice.

Finally, it has shortened the average duration of disease, diminished the expense of treatment enormously, economized the vital resources of the patient, and delivered its friends from the frequently baneful and long-lasting effects of enormous doses of medicine.

In conclusion, I will give a few statistics, from different and reliable authorities; but first, the testimony of Dr. Routh, an eminent Allopathic physician of London, given under circumstances which make it significant and interesting.

In 1852, Dr. Routh published in London a book which he entitled the "Fallacies of

Hom[oe]opathy," which he says he was constrained to do, because

"This system of medical practice has of late unfortunately made, and continues to make, such progress in this country, and the metropolis in particular, and is daily extending its influence even among the most learned, and those whose high positions in society gives them no little moral power over the opinions of the multitude, that our profession is, I think, bound to make it the subject of inquiry and investigation."

To that end, he collected statistics of different hospitals, to the number of thirty-two thousand six hundred and fifty cases, treated in hom[oe]opathic hospitals, and compared them with an equal number of cases from old-school hospitals. He was astonished to find that the average mortality under allopathic treatment was 10.5 per c.; while under hom[oe]opathic treatment it was only 4.4 per c. Still he was honest enough to publish the results. He further states that, proportionally to the number of beds, in hom[oe]opathic hospitals there are twice as many patients admitted and cured, as in allopathic hospitals.

He also states that the mean duration of treatment in pneumonia was

Hom[oe]opathic, 11-2/3 days. Allopathic, 29 days.

After visiting Vienna, Dr. Routh gives the following statistics of cases of inflammation of the lungs, treated respectively in the Hom[oe]opathic and Allopathic Hospitals of that city.

Allopathic mortality 23 per c.

Hom[oe]opathic mortality 5 per c.

Here, then, is allopathic testimony, the most conclusive; that, in this fatal disease, the old system involves a mortality of 23 per c., while that of Hom[oe]opathy is only 5 per c.--just about one-fifth!

I have in my possession, and could adduce here, numerous equally valuable statistics, but as I have already trespassed upon your time, I will sum up the whole in a carefully prepared table of several life insurance companies which have investigated the influence of medical treatment as affecting human life, and from which they feel authorized in offering an annual reduction of 15 per c. to practical hom[oe]opathists. We find the "Atlantic Mutual" making the following deductions:

First. "That practical Hom[oe]opathists enjoy more robust health."

Second. "That they are less frequently attacked by disease."

Third. "When attacked, they recover more rapidly than those treated by any other system."

Fourth. "That the mortality in the more fatal forms of disease is small compared with that under Allopathic treatment."

Fifth. "That many diseases, which are incurable under any other system, are curable under Hom[oe]opathic treatment."

This statement is followed by a general summary from carefully prepared tables, comprising a large mass of statistics, collected from all parts of the world, and embracing the records of the treatment of some 300,000 cases of disease. We find that the ratio of mortality between Hom[oe]opathic and Allopathic treatment, omitting the fractions, to be,--

In General diseases as 4 to 13 " Cholera, as 16 to 49 " Typhus fever, as 8 to 33 " Yellow fever, as 5 to 43 " Pneumonia, as 5 to 31

The general average of all diseases being as 8 to 34, while the average length of sickness under the two systems, is as 2 to 3, a clear gain of over fifty per c. is shown in favor of Hom[oe]opathy.

The inquiry will here naturally arise:--Why is it that, if the Hom[oe]opathic system presents such superior results, that it has not been adopted by the profession generally? While its adherents may with pride refer to its rapid growth in this country, its practitioners having increased from 6 in 1830 to over 6,000 in 1871; yet, if the system is all that its adherents claim, why should it still meet with the most bitter opposition of the old school, instead of that hearty acceptance which its merits would seem to demand?

Before answering this question, let us see how the medical profession, and professors of other branches of science have received the several great discoveries of the last four hundred years.

Copernicus, who taught that the sun is stationary; that the planets revolve around the sun, and that the apparent revolution of the heavens is caused by the rotation of the earth on its axis,--a system now generally received and acknowledged, was persecuted nearly to death. I found, only twenty years ago, a sect of people in Wisconsin, who still disbelieved this great fact, that the earth moves around the sun.

Gallileo, after being converted to the Copernican theory of the revolution of the earth around the sun, and after having improved the telescope of Copernicus, invited his fellow-professors to make these observations with him. They absolutely refused to even look through Gallileo's telescope, and after he had demonstrated to them by actual experiment, that the trifling difference in the falling of two unequal weights is owing only to the resistance of the air, and after making the experiment twice before the eyes of his opposers in dropping two unequal weights from the tower of Pisa, they did not believe it. He also was persecuted through life.

Franklin's electric experiments were received

in like manner. After they had been read before the Royal Society, they were considered worthless, and he earned nothing but ridicule and abuse.

So it was with Fulton, when he was moving upon the Hudson River with his imperfect steamcraft before the eyes of the people; they said it was impossible, and could not be done. Yes, they denied the fact, and declared him insane after he had done it.

Harvey, who discovered and taught that there is an arterial circulation of blood through the human system, was persecuted through life, his professional enemies styling him the "Circulator," a word, in its original Latin, synifying vagabond or quack.

In the light of these facts, it was not surprising that Hahnemann, after the promulgation of his doctrine, meets the same fate, and from that day to the present, the most bitter denunciations have been poured by the Old School, not only upon him, but on all who have adopted, or have investigated his method.

But Time ever rectifies the mistakes of mankind. The value of the discoveries of all these great men has long since been acknowledged by the world; and the day will and must surely arrive, when the little acorn of Truth, planted by Hahnemann, which has already taken deep root, and is lifting high its vigorous stem, shall tower far above all other giants of the medical forest, and its wide-spreading branches cast their beneficent shadows over the whole earth.

F. HILLER, M. D. SAN FRANCISCO, April 10th, 1872. "HOM[oe]OPATHY AND

REGULAR MEDICINE."

The editor of the Buffalo Medical and Surgical Journal (old school) had a sudden spasm of good sense--a condition none too frequent with our Allopathic brethren, and during the attack, allowed the following communication to appear in the pages of his journal.

To the Editor of the Buffalo Medical and Surgical Journal:

It will be to the advantage of the regular medical profession to go carefully over their treatment of the class of physicians who have seen fit to denominate themselves hom[oe]opathic, and to observe the effect such treatment has had upon the profession itself, upon the public and upon hom[oe]opathy.

That the accumulated experience of faithful observers, who, for the last four thousand years have given their lives to the study and treatment of diseases, is, we believe, of almost invaluable importance to one who wishes to become a physician, and certainly is of infinite importance when compared with a hypothetical dogma, and yet, with all the machinery of our hospitals and dispensaries, the control of every medical appointment in the gift of governments or corporations, with our medical schools perfectly equipped with professors for every separate department of medicine, and an entire monopoly of the advantages of clinical observations, with all these advantages and precedents, what headway have we made in convincing the public and individuals of our superior ability to manage disease, or of our peculiar fitness for becoming the sanitary officers of households or communities?

The line of treatment which the regular profession saw fit to adopt in the earliest days of hom[oe]opathy, and which they are still following, is generally bigoted, and universally intolerant opposition. What is the effect of this opposition? It is to arouse in the public mind that generous American sentiment which ever asserts itself to see fair play between a big boy and a little one. There is scarcely an instance in which the regular profession, with all its accumulated prestige, has arrayed itself against hom[oe]opathy, where the weaker party have not prevailed. And to-day, in the sight of the law, and in the confidence of the people, hom[oe]opathy is the peer of regular medicine.

It becomes us to go over this case, and, if possible, discover why, we so strong in numbers, and in all the facilities and appliances for illustrating and inforcing our tenets, are so repeatedly beaten? Why is it that individuals and corporations are becoming convinced that their interests require them to employ hom[oe]opathic in preference to regular physicians? For myself, in spite of the logic of events, I still believe, and my belief is founded upon a thorough investigation of the principles of hom[oe]opathy, and observations upon the practice of many of its most distinguished disciples, that in no way can a man so efficiently equip himself for the responsibility of the management of disease, and the custody of health as in the study of regular medicine.

If we take it for granted that the past experience and observations of physicians are of service to physicians at present, and I do not think we will be charged with assumption for considering this an axiom; then why is it that a sect which disregards all traditions of medicine, and found their system upon a dogma which contradicts all that we have held as truth, why is it that they are flourishing and we are going to the wall?

The answer to this question presents itself to my mind under two heads, which may be formularized as follows: Hom[oe]opathy lives upon the disgrace brought upon the profession of medicine by the low standard of medical education, and flourishes upon the intolerant opposition it has received at the hands of regular physicians.

It is with the second, the lesser of the two evils I propose to deal at this time.

The treatment of hom[oe]opathy by the regular profession in past years is so well known as to require no mention, therefore let us turn our attention to the present, and by reading its signs in the light of the past, endeavor to do something for our future.

The position of the regular profession in regard to hom[oe]opathy may be expressed in a few words. We are not aware of their existence. They have no professional rights which we are bound to respect, and when forced by some laymen to speak upon the subject, or give an opinion upon hom[oe]opathy, the opinion is that it is a "humbug." This line of treatment was bad enough when hom[oe]opathy was young, but now when we stand on equal footing before the law, and nearly equal before the public, it is suicidal.

It may be well to explain what I mean by equal rights before the law. All the rights which members of the regular profession of this State enjoy are granted them by Acts of Legislature, the first of which was passed April 10th, 1813, this and the Act of 1827, contain the "Regulations concerning the Practice of Physic and Surgery in this State." They provide for the establishment of County Medical Societies, "the only organization existing under law for the purpose of diffusing true science and knowledge of the healing art," and otherwise point out and fix the duties, responsibilities and immunities of physicians and surgeons.

On April 13th, 1857, the Legislature of this State admitted the hom[oe]opathic profession to all the rights and privileges enjoyed by members of the regular profession under the above mentioned Acts. This provided for the present, and in the Acts incorporating their colleges, exactly the same power is granted to them as had been granted to our medical schools, which provides for the future. I doubt not there are members of our profession who have hitherto failed to realize the change wrought in the hom[oe]opathic profession by the Acts of 1857. As before stated, the Act admitted the hom[oe]opathic profession to all the rights and privileges as physicians and surgeons under the Acts of 1813 and 1827, and all Acts amendatory thereof, thus they became "legally authorized practicing physicians and surgeons," and as such, are entitled to membership of our County Medical Societies. This right is positive, and no County Society has the power to adopt a by-law which will keep them out if they should make application for admission. The right of legally authorizing physicians to membership of County Medical Societies has been most definitely settled by our courts, and the proceedings to obtain such rights are well understood by many of our members.

In view of these facts what should the regular profession do in the matter? Shall we continue to call ourselves "the profession," and neither by public act or private word allow that there is any other? Shall we continue a line of treatment condemned by law and by experience, treatment which only makes hom[oe]opathy notorious and ourselves disgraceful; or shall we submit gracefully to the laws of the State, and public opinion, and proffer to the hom[oe]opathic profession those amenities which should exist between professional equals? Invite them to the rights in our County Medical Societies, when called by their patrons, attend with them in consultation; when wished by our patients ask them to attend in consultation with us? If they have any superior knowledge in the management of the disease or the protection of health, our duty to our patrons requires us to avail ourselves of that knowledge. If we possess the greater professional ability, they and their patrons will find it out. If we hold back from this, we may reasonably be charged with having little confidence in our doctrines. If we go into it, I rest my faith upon "the survival of the fittest."

Buffalo, August, 1871

H. R. HOPKINS, M. D.

www.ingramcontent.com/pod-product-compliance
Lightning Source LLC
Chambersburg PA
CBHW031444210526
45464CB00005B/2326